5+1=0

Natural Wellness
For
The
Eliminative Pathways

Soulvay Plevell

Copyright © 2016 Amanda Plevell, Soulvay Plevell, The Natural Source

Flight Plan Publishing

All rights reserved.

ISBN- 13: 978-1494857790
ISBN-10: 1494857790

****

To the ladies of the original Natural Source: You have been my friends, my sisters, my counselors, my coaches, my healers and my inspiration. Here's to making a difference, which you all did well every day!

Other books by Soulvay Plevell

(may be published under Amanda Plevell or Soulvay Plevell):

No Grain No Pain

Taking a Break From Crazy

The Love Letters

The Energy of Divorce

Successful Relationships

Mandalas: A Coloring Book

Success Conditioning Journal

Food Functions Nourishment Program

Sneak Chef and The Sugar Free SuperForce

Success Conditioning Work it out Book

I am Success

Gifts of a Dragonfly

Anxiety Turnaround

Tribe

Your Great Big Beautiful Life

Table of Contents

Overview

1. Liver and Bowels
2. Kidney and Bladder
3. Lymphatic and Circulatory
4. Respiratory
5. Skin
6. Emotions

Resources

References

I believe life is very good at bringing us exactly what we need, just when we need it. Interestingly, my body had many spiritual, mental and emotional challenges that all represented themselves physically. At the apex of each physical health challenge, I recognized that the particular challenges and symptoms related to specific systems of the body, if I were to break the body down into six systems: liver and bowels, kidney and bladder, lymphatic and circulation, lung and respiratory, skin, and mind and emotions. Interestingly, I seemed to go through challenges in EACH of these six areas, in the succession that I wrote above. I went from major disasters in my physical health, and as my body healed, it seemed to do so in the above order of systems. While I too make use of other means of health care, I prefer a naturopathic, natural, and holistic path whenever possible. It is my belief not to try to "heal" the symptoms of the body, but to remove the interferences that keep the body responding in acts of illness and instead allow the body to return to a state of peace, and happiness, with the result being health.

What is contained in this book is basically a collection of resources I found and notes from my journal of the research I found for myself and what I did through diet, supplementation and lifestyle changes. I am publishing it in print with the intention that perhaps others are going through what I went through and I could save them some time and pain if they related. While this book is not intended as medical advice and should not be taken as if it were a prescription or direction for health, I hope it gives you some considerations for you and your provider to use for your own body's wellness. As a wellness practitioner, I have enjoyed sharing experiences with clients, but there again, none of this experience qualifies me to tell you specifically what to do through writing a book, and you reading it. This is my research, what I used for myself, and my thoughts and opinions. Be smart and educate yourself and talk to the providers you trust.

As I do not get the opportunity to meet with each one of you individually, I cannot and do not make any guarantees about your abilities to get results with these opinions, ideas, tools, or strategies. Nothing in this book or any resource listed is a promise or guarantee of results and I do not offer any medical or otherwise professional advice. Your results are up to you. My intention is to serve you by sharing what I have gleaned from the numerous books, classes, and strategies I have employed over the years. My intention is a mission of service. I am assuming that your intention is also only for the good and trust that you are using common sense in ALL information that you come across to deem what is or is not appropriate for you and that you are looking to your intelligence and your medical advisors for any help that you need.

Yours in health,

Soulvay Plevell

OVERVIEW

In this day and age, opportunities are plentiful to feel stressed about the body condition or the feeling that something isn't "quite right".

It feels stressful to get down to the nitty gritty and determine "what's wrong" with the body, often sending us on a whirlwind of doctors' appointments, drugs and experimental methods.

The number of diseases has never been greater, the need for medical staff never higher, and the amount of money spent on pharmaceuticals and over the counter drugs never as profitable as it is currently.

I preface this writing by stating that if you feel you have an acute, medical condition, then you should by all means seek the help of an educated professional. Nothing you read in this or any book, website, email, newsletter, or the like should substitute for expert medical advice.

Please use the information contained herein as a general overview of successful supports for each eliminative system of the human body, and not as a substitute for an expert medical appointment.

Having said that, it is my opinion that there is a wealth of knowledge and lifestyle choices that we may employ EVERY DAY that help to support our overall health and balance.

We forget that we are in charge of our own health. We cannot live vicariously and frivolously and then expect a drug, a surgery, or a medical doctor to put us back together.

In the vast numbers of clients I have seen, there is one thing that stands out as a highly impactful avenue for keeping the body healthy: the eliminative systems of the body.

In my humble opinion, I feel that no matter WHAT is going on with the body, as long as it has open channels to work itself OUT, there is no reason the body cannot heal! If things can get OUT and you rebuild with things the body needs, then health becomes easy.

This book is dedicated to each of the 5 eliminative systems of the body:
Lymphatic and Circulatory
Liver and Bowels
Kidney and Bladder
Respiratory
Skin

In it are suggestions, thoughts, and ideas of things YOU CAN DO today to support, rebuild, and cleanse each of these imperative systems.

The information presented is my understanding of the working of the systems of the body, surely from a mechanical, functional perspective. My work history and education has afforded me some understanding of the above. However, my study also constitutes a practice of knowledge stemming from a metaphysical perspective. As a medical intuit and visionary, a large part of the work that I do with the human body comes from the picture I have been given of the human body as an energy, not just an entity. This is a major drawback in the field of science and proof, I would say, that limits us to only seeing the physical body that we can touch, monitor, and record, rather than the innerworkings that understanding the body parts as energy brings me. As a visionary and intuit, I can see and feel the parts of the body in form, but also as an energy, seeing sometimes patterns and shifts, vibrations and waves, and often felt as heat and cool, colors and emotion. Seeing the body in this way helps me to see what the part needs or is lacking and why it isn't "playing nice" with the rest of the parts. See, the body is a community. In this community, they don't often know what each other is doing, because they mind their own business. They are so intent on each their own job that they just busily get on doing it, knowing, expecting, and assuming that each will do this. It is my personal opinion that having no interference from the outside world and even our own thoughts, emotions, and actions, they would each continue acting out their parts.

Understanding this, if you find yourself with a symptom or illness, try not to see the symptom or illness, and certainly don't see it as "bad" and hateful. Rather see it openly and love it as you do your child, and compassionately ask what it needs. Try to understand the behavior behind it. See it as separate, discover its properties, and learn what it does best. If you see each part of you with love, it is easier to be compassionate towards yourself, which in turn brings about less stress, and less analytical thought and fear based action. Instead, you are simply allowing the body to speak to you. And through this conversation you are going to find your answer. One of my professors once said, "If you let someone speak long enough, eventually they will tell you what's wrong with them." I believe this is true of the energetic conference in which you can engage your body.

Whether or not you believe what I believe doesn't matter as far as this book is concerned. This book is instructive on the systems of elimination and the belief that it is a major determining factor in the health of the body as a whole.

Imagine a highway with 4 lanes of traffic. What happens when there is an accident and it jams 2 lanes of traffic? Traffic slows and it now doubles your drive time, right? This is true of the eliminative systems of the body. If there are 5 pathways to begin with, but 1, 2, or more are congested, it puts much more pressure on the other pathways to perform and take care of all the "traffic".

If the eliminative systems are working THERE WILL BE HEALTH.

Use this information wisely, and seek your local expert with any questions you may have. The back of the book has resources available to you.

1 LIVER AND BOWEL

Description
Support Activities
Toxins to Avoid
Common Nutritional Supplementation
Foods to Consider
Additional Suggestions

Description

There is an order to everything in nature. It would only make sense that it would be this way within and surrounding our physical bodies. All is well with health if the body can one: intake, and two: output. The eliminative systems are the basis for this output system. What the body is done with, made use of, or is toxic to the body and needs to come out, is what will be flushed through the eliminative systems. It is necessary that all systems are considered as you are focusing on one system of elimination, particularly the first and foremost system: the Liver and Bowels. This is the body's largest line of defense. In order to encourage ANY system of elimination, it helps to make sure this one is clearing, or the toxic effects of elimination would be noticed through the other channels. For example, more pressure would be put on the skin and you could notice rashes, or the lymph system would get sluggish and you would notice a weakened immune system, clogged lymph nodes or skin rash.

It is unequivocally important to make sure this system is working, for health of the entire body.

There are some methods that I use quite frequently to assist this function.

* Daily I eat well, at least juicing daily if nothing else.
* I eliminate and keep out of my diet anything that does not comprise a good nourishment foundation, like pop, caffeine, sugars and processed foods.
* I eliminate any foods that I know cause allergies or intolerances.
* In addition to this DAILY care, WEEKLY I fast or cleanse through the form of a liquid diet or juicing all day, for one single day. I ensure I am getting plenty of water, as well as juicing all the fruits and vegetables that I consume that day. It is as simple weekly detox.
* Yearly, I do quarterly detoxes that involve elimination of certain foods for a longer period of time, (usually a week to 21 days). There are a

number of programs that do 21 day detoxes and your natural health provider can help you find the right one for you. There is the sugar detox, detox challenges through companies like Melaleuca, Genesis Pure, Metagenics, Kannaway, The Inner Klean Diet from Dr. Thurman Fleet, and many more. It basically is a change for the body, out of the usual style of eating it is used to. Just switching up your eating can and will detox the body. If I am going to do supplemental detoxifiers or cleanses, now is the time that I use these. Otherwise, all year long it is simply done with food.

* I use coffee enemas and swear by them! If the body is ill, if the body is mucosal, if the body has skin problems, I use coffee enemas! These are a gentle, fantastic, effective way to eliminate what the body has not. It keeps the channels clear for elimination and is especially useful, in my opinion, in situations with inflammatory bowel conditions, when the intestines aren't eliminating properly. In my opinion, these enemas can do the job until the intestines can get back to it. There is a wealth of knowledge about coffee enemas. What I use is included in this book.

There are a variety of other enemas that I use also to help heal this sensitive and very important lining. Without health in the gut, you won't find health elsewhere.

HERBAL ENEMAS
Flaxseed tea enemas are known to relieve inflammation in the bowel.
Slippery Elm, marshmallow root, and comfrey are known to be mucosal, healing up the sensitive lining, as well as antimicrobial, as well as being anti-iinfammatory,
For myself, I use a tsp of the powdered herb in 2 c of water and simmer for 15 minutes. Straining it first, I add it to the enema bag.

JUICE FASTING
I believe the rest you give your body just from the demanding exercise of eating all day every day allows it the opportunity to reverse disease processes and recover your health. It's the rest from food and the simple diet that does the trick. The lack of too many food mixtures and less demand made on our digestive and eliminative systems help us to increase health.

THE MASTER CHLOROPHYLL ELIMINATION DIET
There are a great many diets and cleanses out there, and of this, I am wary. Consulting with a professional is highly recommended. I also however, believe in consistent consumption of greens in the diet. With greens in the body, elimination of any mucosal condition is almost inevitable, on a nutrition level. This is a diet of just plain water, preferably using distilled water, and using one teaspoon of a liquid chlorophyll to one glass of water

every three hours. I have also done this by steaming greens, and then drinking the water. This is a diet where we are adding iron from the greens. This iron helps move oxygen through the blood, which burns up toxic material.

Liquid Chlorophyll can be made from extracting alfalfa leaves if you have a good juicer and a hydraulic press, as the majority of the beneficial liquids need an additional pressing after the initial juicing. Alfalfa leaves are one of the best foods for potassium iron.

These liquids can be used daily in addition to a regular diet. Though at times, I will drink only this green juice for a day or so, especially when ill and I need to drink liquids.

VITAL BROTH RECIPE:

This is a vegetable beverage made which retains nutrients for easy consumption and absorption in the body.. It can be added into a diet, as well as using during illness when a liquid diet is recommended.

2 C. carrot tops;
1 clove garlic;
2 C. potato peelings (1/2 thick);
2 C. beet tops;
2 C. celery tops;
3 C. celery stalk;
2 qt distilled water;
Add a carrot and onion to flavor, if desired (grate or chop).
Ingredients should be finely chopped. Bring to a boil, slowly: simmer approximately 20 minutes. Use only the broth after straining.

SUCCESSFUL BOWEL MANAGEMENT THROUGH EXERCISES

I love what Dr. Bernard Jensen has to say for a bowel exercise program. He is a foremost authority on bowel health and has many resources. We don't often think to exercise internal muscles, tendons, and tissues. He makes it apparent how necessary it is.

"A successful bowel management program requires that we go a different way. In following a program for the bowel, there are some excellent corrective exercises. There is an exercise to use on the slant board which involves vigorous tapping of the abdomen while stretching the upper torso from side to side. This exercise gently pulls the bowel down in the direction of the shoulders while upside-down on the board. I'm interested in getting the bowel in the preferred position. I believe we have been crowding the bowel. So we must go to work on it. Doing the bicycle pedaling exercise while up-side down on the slant board is a wonderful exer-cise. For another type of exercise, lie down and take a rubber ball or tennis ball and rub it around in a circle on your abdomen. The round surface of the ball gets right down into the bowel and gives it an internal exercise, more so than rubbing on the outside. There are other exercises to lift the bowel and manipulate the prolapsus back into position.constipation is present."[1]

SUPPLEMENTATION TO LOOK INTO FOR SUPPORT
Bromelain
Feverfew
White willow
Boswellia
Vit c
Turmeric
Vitamin E
Antioxidants
Milk thistle
Dandelion root
Silymarin
Quercetin
Detox teas that contain milk thistle, dandelion root, burdock
Red Rice Yeast Extract (can cause a flushing effect at first)
Especially for intestines: probiotics are essential! Particularly those bacterias of bifidobacterium, lactobacillus, acidophilus. You may have to start one at a time, and try powders so you can adjust the dose. Many can only do small amounts of acidophilus only when they begin probiotic supplementation.
Enzymes - Digestive enzymes, and a full spectrum one at that, are necessary to reduce the amount of digestion that happens in the gut.

*please check with your provider which are appropriate for you. Remember, not all doctors are the same. Find someone who is well -versed in naturopathic or herbal supplementation.

---

[1] Referneces: Dr Schulzes incurables Bernard Jensen

FOODS TO AVOID
Alcohol of all kinds, wine in moderation occasionally or not at all
Sugars
High fat foods
Fried foods
Processed foods
Foods containing dyes, artificial sweeteners, and preservatives.

As the liver is the primary filter for all that comes into the body, it is necessary to look at all he unnatural foods that the liver will have to clear. If it is a product unknown to nature, how will the liver fare over time?

Also, consider the impact of pharmaceuticals and over the counter drugs on the liver. Once again, as primary filter, it is responsible for handling the wastes and the byproducts after the body is done with a certain substance. ALL drugs have a heavy impact on the liver, but some more so than others. Check with your pharmacist and work with your provider to help you use any natural means possible. These include diets, herbs, supplements, and lifestyle changes. You may have to see multiple practitioners, as not all practitioners and doctors are well versed in these. Find people that will combine into a joint effort for your health.

Reduction or elimination of Omega 6 family of fatty acids, which are known to trigger inflammation. These are foods like unhealthy fats and fried foods.

FOODS TO ADD
Omega 3's from supplements or fish oils, or quality sources like Salmon are antiinflammatory in nature by blocking inflammatory cytokines in the body. They also block a certain enzyme that breaks down joint cartilage.
Herbs to season your foods with instead of salts
Bitter greens. Our bodies are bitter in nature and prefer a diet that includes bitters like digestive bitters, bitter greens like kale, arugla, and dandelion greens.
Dandelion root tea which you can make from the root itself, or buy premade.
Ginger
Garlic
Onions
Rosemary
Antioxidant and Vitamin C rich sources like berries and citrus

Probiotic foods like kefir, yogurt(particularly homemade yogurt), kombucha, fermented vegetables, homemade sauerkraut
Quality fat sources like avocado and nuts.

*Keep in mind, these are general suggestions and in no way suggest they are suitable to all bodies.

ADDITIONAL SUGGESTIONS
Visceral massage
Craniosacral work
* It has been noticed that women will experience IBS or a worsening of IBS symptoms during their menstrual period. "In one trial, women with IBS who experienced worsening symptoms before and during their menstrual period were helped by taking evening primrose oil."[2] Borage seed oil, black currant seed oil, and flax oil are others to try.

---

[2] Dr. Schulze's Incurables

CASTOR OIL PACKS
(per wellnessmama.com)

Castor oil packs have been said to help improve liver detoxification naturally, support uterine and ovarian health, improve lymphatic circulation and reduce inflammation.

The idea is to keep castor oil on a piece of cloth on the skin for at least an hour with a heat source to stimulate lymph and liver function. Unlike some "detox" methods, this is not said to have any negative side effects and the there are many accounts of people who noticed immediate better sleep, more energy and clearing of skin symptoms.

There aren't any conclusive studies on the use of castor oil packs externally (though there are some preliminary ones), but a long history of traditional use in many cultures. There is some evidence that it can have a suppressive effect on tumors and a positive effect on arthritis when used externally. Castor oil packs also provide time of quiet relaxation, which also has health benefits, so I thought they were worth a try.

Castor oil packs have traditionally been used on various body parts:

- On the right side of the abdomen or the whole abdomen, which is thought to help support the liver and digestive system
- On strained joints or muscles (not as a substitute for medical care but to speed healing of minor injuries that don't need medical attention)
- On the lower abdomen to help with menstrual pain and difficulties

Even for external use, I'd consult with a doctor or naturopath to make sure that this natural remedy is ok for you. It should not be used if pregnant or struggling with a medical condition. I also test any new oil (or any substance) on a small part of my arm before using on a larger area of the body.

How to Do a Castor Oil Pack

Castor oil packs are simple to do at home and I like them because they require me to be still and relax and read a book for at least an hour. They can be messy, but with proper preparation are not.

Needed Supplies

- High-quality castor oil (hexane free) – I've gotten from Radiant Life Catalog and Mountain Rose Herbs
- Unbleached and dye free wool or cotton flannel (like this)- can be reused up to 30 times
- A wrap around pack (plastic free) or plastic wrap (not optimal)
- Hot water bottle or heating pad
- Glass container with lid – I use a quart size mason jar (for storing the oil soaked flannel between uses)
- Old clothes, towels and sheets – castor oil does stain
- Patience (most difficult to find!)

The easiest and least messy option I've found is the Castor Oil Pack kit from here. It has the castor oil, cotton flannel and a non-messy wrap around pack that removes the need for plastic wrap and has kept mine from leaking at all.

How to Do A Castor Oil Pack

I highly recommend carefully prepping the area where you'll be doing the castor oil pack to prevent mess. I like using an old shower curtain, covered with a sheet under me, just to make sure nothing stains. I don't often have to wash the sheet, and I just fold and store in the bathroom cabinet for the next use.

Before Beginning:

- Cut a large piece of cotton flannel and fold into thirds to make three layers. My original piece was 20 inches by 10 inches and when folded it was roughly 7×10 but yours could be larger or smaller, depending on where you are planning to place it.
- Thoroughly soak (but not completely saturate) the flannel in castor oil. The easiest way I found to do this was to carefully fold the

flannel and place in a quart size mason jar. I then added castor oil about a tablespoon at a time (every 20 minutes or so) to give it time to saturate. I also gently shook the jar between adding more oil so that the oil could reach all parts of the cloth. Ideally, this should be done the day before to give it time to evenly soak. I save the jar since this is where I keep the flannel between uses (it can be used about 30 times).

Using a Castor Oil Pack:

1. Carefully remove and unfold the castor oil soaked cloth.
2. While lying on an old towel or sheet, place the cloth on the desired body part.
3. Cover with plastic (like a plastic trash bag), or ideally with the wrap around pack, and place the heating pack on top of this. A hot water bottle, electric heating pad or rice heating pad can be used, but hot water bottles and rice packs may need to be reheated several times.
4. Lie on back with feet elevated (I typically lie on the floor and rest my feet on the couch), and relax for 30-60 minutes.
5. Use this time to practice deep breathing, read a book, meditate or pray (or whatever you find relaxing).
6. After the desired time, remove the pack and return the flannel to the glass container. Store in fridge.
7. Use a natural soap or a mix of baking soda and water to remove any castor oil left on the skin.
8. Relax and rest. Make sure to drink enough water and stay hydrated after doing this.

Other ways to use castor oil:

From Japanese Healing Arts:

Castor oil is used externally in three ways. First, castor oil may be applied directly to the skin for dryness, rashes, hives, fungus, infections, boils, furuncles, liver spots (age spots), warts, benign skin cancers, etc. Also for infection or fungus in the finger or toe nails. Apply castor oil directly and gently rub into the area for a minute or two. Repeat this application 2 or 3 times a day for a few weeks or up to two months in the case of stubborn warts.

Second, the application of castor oil packs can bring significant relief for any kind of trauma, sprain or degenerative joint disorder. In the case of a painful joint, apply a pack and secure it with an ace bandage. Keep the pack on the body continuously and reapply castor oil every 24 hours. For back pain, lay on a castor oil pack for 90 minutes every day for 5 days. (See instructions below.) In severe cases, you may have to repeat this course 3 times over a period of 3 weeks.

Third, castor oil packs are used for cleansing and regulating the internal organs. For disorders relating to the digestion, intestines, liver, lungs or reproductive organs a series of castor oil packs on the abdomen for 90 minutes a day can have remarkable effects.[3]

YOGURT INSTRUCTIONS[4]
The following directions will yield 2 liters of delicious, snuggly, homemade SCD yogurt.
1. Pour 2 litres of milk into a clean pot and heat to at least 180°F, maintaining that temperature for 2 minutes. It is OK if the milk boils. Note: whenever you measure the milk's temperature, be sure to stir the milk for 15-30 seconds to get an overall reading.
2. Allow the milk to cool to below 100°F, or to room temperature. You can speed up the cooling process by putting the pot into a bath of cool water.
3. Pour the cooled milk into the plastic batch jar/container.
4. Pour two packages (10 grams) of starter into a measuring cup, and gradually stir in 5-6 Tablespoons of the cooled milk. Once the starter is completely dissolved, pour it into the remainder of the cooled milk in the batch container. Stir thoroughly. It is essential that the starter and the milk are blended evenly.
5. Cover the batch container with the snap-on lid.
6. Using the marks on the inside of the yogurt maker, pour water to the top of the taller mark ("2 liter marker"). Lower the prepared batch container into the yogurt maker. The water will come up on

---

[3] http://wellnessmama.com/35671/castor-oil-packs/
[4] http://www.scdiet.org/2recipes/scdyogurt.html

the outside of the batch container to the same height as the milk inside. Cover the yogurt maker and plug in the power cord. The red light will come on.
7. Allow the yogurt to ferment for 24 hours. Do not move the yogurt maker during this time.
8. Unplug the yogurt maker and remove the batch container. You are now 8 hours away from delicious yogurt...
9. Gently place the batch container into the refrigerator and chill for 8 hours.
10. The homemade SCD yogurt is ready after chilling for 8 hours. The yogurt will stay fresh for three weeks if kept cold.

Note: do not add gelatin or powdered milk to the yogurt batch (as is suggested in the manufacturer's instruction manual).

COFFEE ENEMAS
Start with an enema kit containing a 2 qt. hot water bag
Recipe 2 qt. distilled water (8 cups)
6 tbsp. Organic (must use organic and with caffeine) ground coffee. Combine coffee with water (distilled) and cover. Bring to a boil, reduce heat to simmer, for 20 min. Strain through coffee filter and wait for coffee to come to room temp or body temp, Do not use with temperature over 101 degrees, (use a thermometer to protect you) fill bag only after checking the temperature. Use some coconut oil to lubricate end and insert no more than 3 inches into bowel. If encountering resistance you're in to far and need to back out some. Using a timer set for 15 minutes from beginning to end, slowly insert small amounts of liquid until the bag is empty. If you can't go the full 15 minutes this is fine but the more time the liquid stays in the body the more it can clean the blood, intestines, and liver. Allow the necessary time for everything to come out of the colon. You may be sitting on the toilet for sometime. Do not force anything, but allow the peristaltic action to take place. Be close to toilet the whole time as there is not a lot of time to make it if too far away. Lying is the best recommendation and being completely comfortable while lying down using towels under you can create comfort. Use something that can be easily washed. There are several positions one can take in administering the liquid, but the most beneficial is just laying on your back. For achieving dramatic results do this cleanse for 7 days twice daily, Am and Pm. If you are not used to caffeine you can do the second cleanse of the day using a decaffeinated organic coffee. You may feel as if you need to periodically do a cleanse as a once a month method as you repair your body through nutritional means. This will slow to a point of nonexistence or on a once a month maintenance practice of a 1 time cleanse am or pm to keep things moving through.

Remember while you do the 7 days or even while doing a 1 day cleanse throughout the month you should take supplements to replenish the electrolytes. Electrolytes are Magnesium, Potassium, Calcium, Chloride and Sodium. These can be easily supplied by drinking a good coconut water. Also drink good clean water in one hour intervals to make sure you are putting back the moisture that will be lost. If you have a tendency to forget to drink you should set a timer for 1 hour intervals, each time drinking at least 4 to 6 oz. of good clean water (not city water unless filtered). Make sure you pay close attention to clean up and use a good sanitizing cleanser or hydrogen peroxide to clean up any feces. Also used to clean the bag and the insertion tube.[5]

DIETS

Eating a particular diet that is specific to anti-inflammation is key in keeping the intestines whole and intact, healthy, and prepared to absorb nutrients without breakdown and the creation of Leaky Gut Syndrome. Popular diets in this category almost always eliminate most if not all grains and sugars. These include: The AutoImmune Protocol, No grain No Pain, SCD, Paleo. Quality resources are listed in the resource section in the back of this book.

Sometimes a basic anti-inflammatory diet is not enough and the body needs to go further in it's healing. This sometimes means avoiding nightshades, like tomatoes, potatoes, eggplants, sweet and hot peppers, and chili based spices. In this case, I follow a anti-inflammatory diet along with avoidance of nightshades.

"Nightshades can be problematic for many people due to their lectin, saponin and/or capsaicin content. They tend to be even more problematic for those with autoimmune disease and of all the foods restricted in the autoimmune protocol, are probably the least likely to be successfully reintroduced, especially tomatoes and chilies. There are over 2000 plant species in the nightshade family, the vast majority of which are inedible and many are highly poisonous (like deadly nightshade and jimsomweed). Tobacco is also a nightshade, and is known to cause heart, lung, and circulatory problems as well as cancer and other health problems (clearly some of this has to do with the other toxins in tobacco products derived from the processing). Of the edible species in the nightshade family, poisoning can actually occur with excessive consumption and it is possible

---

[5] Recipe courtesy of Kelli Spencer and Dr. Schulze's Incurables

that the low-level toxic properties of the nightshade vegetables contribute to a variety of health issues as they progress over time."[6]

Certain foods damage a body based on their ability to break them down, and how they are used by the body. One potentially problematic food for a sensitive gut are lectins. "The lectins which we avoid in the paleo diet are the ones with the ability to increase intestinal impermeability. These are lectins which resist digestion ….have the ability to strongly interact with proteins in the membrane of the cells that line the intestine."[7]

Phenolic Therapy
There are times when a system has become so unbalanced and incapable of handling digestion, that a process called Phenolic Therapy is used. It is my premise that sometimes it is not the whole food itself that is causing the problem, but the chemicals that the food breaks down into once ingested into the body. As this is my own research, I am happy to answer questions on this theory if you email me directly.

While only touching on the subject, the above measures are my "go to" items when I think of any autoimmune response.

---

[6] The WHYs behind the Autoimmune Protocol: Nightshades Foods in Moderation, The WHYs of the AIP by ThePaleoMom
[7] ThePaleoMom

2 KIDNEY AND BLADDER
Description
Support Activities
Toxins to Avoid
Common Nutritional Supplementation
Foods to Consider
Additional Suggestions

Description

The kidneys are one of the biggest filters for the body, besides the liver. All 5 physical eliminative systems are necessary and the kidneys and bladder are second in the line of defense. As you work on any of the other eliminative systems. It is wise to make sure the colon is processing wastes and the kidneys are processing fluids. Otherwise a back up in these areas can be very painful and risky to health.

Support Activities

Visceral massage helps keep the internal abdominal organs toned and healthy.

Kegel exercises are useful in keeping internal muscles strong and bladder and urethra firm. This is for men and women.

Common Sense Urination, going to the bathroom at the first tinge, rather than holding it. There is a misguided belief that holding your urine will strengthen your bladder, when I believe it really just creates time for bacteria to develop.

This is especially true in children that are potty training and elderly that are using adult diapers. Both groups need to be reminded to use the bathroom in a timely manner.

Castor oil packs can be used with the same method as for the liver, and placed on the back over the kidneys.

Hydration includes not only intake of pure water, but electrolyte and mineral containing water like coconut water. A common measurement to insure you are intaking enough water is consider getting about half your body weight in ounces of water per day. For example, if I weigh 100 lbs, I would drink about 50 oz in water.

Toxins to Avoid

As for all of the eliminative systems, and as a major filtering system for the body, it is important to avoid ingested and environmental toxins. As much as you can do so, the less your body will have to fight. This includes low VOC paints and stains, alternative flooring options, and possibly buying used rather than new to reduce off gassing.

Metals and the poisoning that comes from heavy metals is especially important to the kidneys, as well as any contaminants that travel through the bloodstream. The use of tobacco is not only a concern for the lungs, but the cadmium that is found in tobacco can be a contributor to renal insufficiency.[8]

Supplements to Consider:
Rhubarb
Chitosan
Coenzyme Q-10
Astragalus
Antioxidants

You will want to discuss supplemental and food choices with your provider, as some supplements and foods can worsen the condition, and/or contribute to kidney stones as an indirect action of the food or supplements.

Foods to Consider
Some of the best kidney supports and detoxifiers:

Parsley water is my favorite. Parsley has been said to be able to break up kidney stones. You simply boil a handful of fresh parsley in water and drink throughout the day.

Cucumbers are a natural diuretic. I drink cucumber juiced alongside parsley, carrot, apple, celery every morning. I believe it to be a natural daily nutritional effort to keeping the kidneys healthy as well as the bladder. One other benefit: the cucumber has a nice slippery mucosal quality that can prevent bacteria from adhering to the lining of the bladder.

---

[8] https://www.merckmanuals.com/professional/genitourinary-disorders/tubulointerstitial-diseases/heavy-metal-nephropathy

Detox tea has pau d'arco in it which is soothing and gentle to the body in a slowly detoxifying way. Pau D'arco is known for it's benefit to the bladder.

Cranberry is a first go to nutritional product to support the kidneys. I am wary of using cranberry juice, however, for its sugar content and potential for the sugar to feed any present bacteria, causing UTI, bladder, and kidney infections. I use Azo cranberry over the counter in a pinch, or boil fresh or frozen cranberries and drink the liquid.

Oregano oil and garlic are known natural antibiotics. Taken internally, they can help support the body's immune system when in need.

Goldenseal and Myrrh herbal tinctures are a wonderful gentler concoction with natural antibiotic properties.

Drinking vegetable broth helps to keep the kidneys flushed, as well as making sure to stay hydrated with fresh pure water.

I always use probiotics to support a healthy balance of gut microflora.

When doing any lymphatic or skin work, I make sure to support the kidneys so there isn't backup in detoxification. Any elimination work that I do I make sure to do coffee enemas as they can help the body remove more toxins.

1 Tbsp Apple cider vinegar with 1 tbsp honey is a powerful combination to kill bacteria that could be present.
Aloe vera juice is a great nutritional help, as well as marshmallow root, ginger, and milk thistle.[9]

Urinary Tract/Bladder Infection Relief of Symptoms
*from author's own journal

---

[9] *Please understand these are notes from my own personal care and should be used for educational purposes only. I am not a medical doctor and cannot diagnose, treat, heal, cure, or prescribe. Please talk to your health care provider.

The following has been known to help the symptoms of infections of the bladder and urinary tract. These are the author's experiences. I am sharing what I have done and do for myself when in that situation.

I supplement with:
1 Tbsp colloidal silver, 3 times a day
5 drops oregano oil, straight into throat followed by 1 cup of milk, soymilk, hempmilk, or coconut milk, then a glass of water
Lots of water throughout the day, to flush the bacteria from the tissue
1 clove of garlic, chopped, and swallowed with water 3 times a day
Use colloidal silver on a clean piece of toilet paper to wipe front to back
1000mg Vitamin C once daily
capsules of Azo Cranberry, bought over the counter. Not all cranberry products are the same. I do not drink cranberry juice at this time as the sugar of the juice may actually worsen the problem
D- Mannose prevents the bacteria from sticking to the lining, bought at a natural foods store

I eat:
Mostly a liquid diet as I want my body's energy to be used to fight the infection
Lots of water and clear fluids
Bone Broth made with chicken and vegetables
No sugar, grains, bread, rice or noodle products
Cooked vegetables
*Sugar feeds the bacteria or yeast, and grains break down into sugar

Other tips:
I do coffee enemas at this time. The release of bowels helps to rid the body of toxins, as well as lightening pressure in the abdomen
I use light warm heating pads to the lower abdomen and pelvis for comfort
I do not take OTC medications or prescription medications that block the pain, burn, or urgency. My thought is the body is trying to eradicate the bacteria from the body and it does that through frequent urination. Take a me day, grab a book and some movies and hang out in the bathroom so you can go whenever you feel the urge.
I take epsom salt and apple cider vinegar baths. I pour 1 cup epsom salt and ¼ cup apple cider vinegar in as the water is running. This soothes and cleanses

If these methods are applied at the first signs, the symptoms are relieved in the day. I continue to take the supplements and healthy measures for a week to 2 weeks following.[10]

Help for Overworked Kidneys (according to Swanson Vitamins.com)

Six supplements offer significant help for your kidneys as detailed below. Keep in mind however, like most systems of the body, the kidneys really respond best to a healthy diet that includes plenty of fruits and vegetables plus 8 glasses of pure water.

1. Aloe Vera Juice—Aloe is very cleansing to the body, and the kidneys love it! Mix up a health cocktail from the juice of one squeezed lemon, an ounce of aloe vera juice, 6 ounces of bottled water and a teaspoon of honey (for sweetening) to keep the kidneys performing at their very best. Lemon juice and aloe vera provide noteworthy levels of citric acid or citrate. When citrate binds to calcium, it prevents this mineral from massing together to form stones.
2. Vitamin B-6—Helps prevent the formation of calcium oxalate.
3. Magnesium—Lowers urinary oxalate, which is a mineral salt.
4. Uva Ursi— Herbal support that benefits the entire urinary tract including the kidneys, bladder and urethra.

---

[10] I am not a medical doctor. I cannot and do not diagnose, cure, treat, heal, or prescribe.
Please see qualifying health provider for your particular concerns
Use the following information for educational purposes

5. Parsley—Increases the flow of urine, thereby assisting the kidneys to flush the body of wastes.
6. Chlorella—Helps maintain an alkaline environment in which the kidneys thrive.

Please remember that I am not a medical doctor and cannot diagnose, heal, treat, cure, or prescribe.

3 Lymphatics and Circulatory

Description
Support Activities
Toxins to Avoid
Common Nutritional Supplementation
Foods to Consider
Additional Suggestions

Description

The body has two circulatory systems: Lymphatic and blood.

The circulatory systems of the body are meant to circulate oxygen, and nutrients throughout the body, and then to carry waste products or harmful bacterias and toxins out.

Essentially, the lymphatic system is your first circulatory system. It's job is to collect all the waste from the cellular fluid around the cells. This fluid swims in and through cells and also around the cells. This fluid allows nutrients to be carried into the cells and allows cells to release wastes and carry them out of the body.

This all happens in lymphatic fluid. This fluid now cycles AROUND the organs until it is in the lymph nodes at the throat which can then be released, swallowed, and processed through the eliminative pathways of kidney and liver.

We want lymphatic to do it's job. If it does not, it puts more pressure on the blood circulatory system to take care of it all. The main difference is that the blood system goes to ALL OF THE ORGANS.

Now, the blood system has a pump to continuously push it's fluid through: the heart.

Lymphatic system does not have a pump. The only way it moves is if YOU move. Cardio exercise is great for blood circulatory, but does not necessarily move the lymphatic.

Support Activities
Lymphatic bounce exercises on a large exercise ball. Let your body move with the bounce.

Trampoline -
One great thing you can easily do is purchase a mini trampoline and bounce or jump for just fifteen minutes a day.

If you are at risk of knee, back, or joint injury, please content yourself with a mild bouncing without lifting your feet off of the trampoline.

Swinging -is also a great activity to stimulate the lymphatic system.

Dry Skin Brushing - see following directions.

Oil Pulling

Lymphatic massage

DRY SKIN BRUSHING
(according to www.livestrong.com)

Dry skin brushing is a simple technique whereby the lymphatic pathways are stimulated by the gentle massage and guidance of the outer layer of the skin, triggering the nerves that affect the lymph nodes. Dry skin brushing done properly helps to stimulate lymphatic flow

How to Dry Skin Brush:

Dry skin brushing has been practiced for thousands of years. The Japanese brushed their skin before their traditional hot bath. Ancient Greek athletes used spoon-like scrapers to remove grime and stimulate circulation. The Cherokee Indians used dried corn cobs to brush their skin to enhance beauty and durability. The Comanche Indians used sand from the Texas river bottoms to scrub their skin. Dry skin brushing exfoliates and stimulates new skin growth. It cleanses the lymphatic system, removes dead skin and cellulite, tightens skin, tones muscles and stimulates circulation.

It's easy once you get the hang of it, and it only takes 15 minutes to your entire body.

Step 1

Dry brush your skin first in the morning, before you shower. Start from the feet or head, whichever you prefer. Your skin should be completely dry. If starting from the feet, brush the feet in a circular motion. Brush your legs using upward strokes and your arms using upward strokes from the hands. Brush your torso in an upward motion and your stomach in a circular motion. Lightly brush your breasts in a circular motion. Brush your back from the base of your neck down the tailbone as far as you can reach. Use more vigorous strokes on areas where your skin is thick--like your soles, and light strokes on areas where your skin is thin. Don't brush irritated or broken skin.

Step 2

Dry brush once a day, first thing in the morning. You can brush areas with cellulite twice a day for about five to 10 minutes to minimize the appearance of cellulite. Do this consistently for five months for best results.

Step 3

Take a three-minute hot shower after you are finished dry brushing, followed with a 10- to 20-second cold rinse. Repeat this hot-and-cold shower three times. You may substitute a warm shower if you can take the hot-and-cold showers. This invigorates and stimulates blood circulation to the skin. Rub the skin down with a loofah sponge to remove dead skin. Dry off and massage the skin with olive, almond or coconut oil to moisturize and soften.

Step 4

Wash your brush with soap and water once a week. Leave it a sunny open area to dry to avoid mildew. Make sure it is dry before brushing the skin.

Step 5

Brush your skin for at least three months to thoroughly cleanse the lymphatic system and achieve the best results. Any new regimen requires time to show results, so be patient and remain consistent with your brushing schedule.[11]

Things You'll Need:

Brush with soft natural bristles and a long handle

Loofah sponge

Olive, avocado, apricot, almond, sesame or coconut oil or cocoa butter

OIL PULLING
(according to www.oilpulling.com)

Oil pulling is simple, in expensive and non invasive.

It's health benefits immediately affect dental and oral health with whiter teeth, fresher breath, and less risk of cavity or infection.

Because the method involves swishing action and vibrates around and near important lymph nodes in the lymphatic system, it is easy to pull toxin from the lymph and waste it through the digestive passage as normal. Like attracts like and the smooth fattiness of the sunflower oil or coconut oil resembles the thick and lubricative mucosal phlegm that is gathered from sinuses, respiration, and lymph nodes.

---

[11] (reference:http://www.livestrong.com/article/184493-how-to-dry-brush-your-skin/)

How to do oil pulling:

"In the morning, before breakfast on an empty stomach you take one tablespoon in the mouth but do not swallow it. Move Oil Slowly in the mouth as rinsing or swishing and Dr Karach puts it as ' sip, suck and pull through the teeth' for fifteen to twenty minutes. This process makes oil thoroughly mixed with saliva. Swishing activates the enzymes and the enzymes draw toxins out of the blood. The oil must not be swallowed, for it has become toxic. As the process continues, the oil gets thinner and white. If the oil is still yellow, it has not been pulled long enough. It is then spit from the mouth , the oral cavity must be thoroughly rinsed and mouth must be washed thoroughly. Just use normal tap water and good old fingers to clean.

Clean the sink properly, you can use some antibacterial soap to clean the sink. Because the spittle contains harmful bacteria and toxic bodily waste. If one were to see one drop of this liquid magnified 600 times under a microscope, one would see microbes in their first stage of development.

It is important to understand that during the oilpulling / oilswishing process one's metabolism is intensified. This leads to improved health. One of the most striking results of this process is the fastening of loose teeth, the elimination of bleeding gums and the visible whitening of the teeth.

The oil pulling /swishing is done best before breakfast. To accelerate the healing process, it can be repeated three times a day, but always before meals on an empty stomach."[12]

TOXINS TO AVOID

---

[12] (reference: http://www.oilpulling.com/)

Because the circulatory system's job is bringing in new oxygen, and new nutrients, as well as "garbage collection", removing or reducing toxins used is an important step for lymphatic and circulatory health.

Heavy metals and chemicals to avoid:

Aluminum found in deodorants, baking powder, toothpastes, aluminum foil and cookware, pop cans

Mercury – dental fillings, air pollution, tattoo ink, hair dye

Cadmium – art supplies, cigarettes, plastics, batteries

Chemicals to avoid:

Acetone

Chlorine

Formaldehyde (found in no iron shirts)

Methylethl Ketone

Pesticides on fruits and vegetables unless organically grown

DDT

Diazinon

Malathion[13]

NUTRITIONAL SUPPLEMENTATION TO CONSIDER:

Colloidal silver will help to prevent bacterial infections

Vitamin A boosts the immune system

---

[13] (reference: Baker, Joyce, *Computerized Electrodermal Screening*", p.24)

Proteus homeopathic – common use in sinus infections

Pyrogenium – sinus infections with green or yellow discharge

Candida and/or fungal remedies

Protease - protein digestion

Copper/gold/silver – antibacterial, anti viral, prone to staph and strep infections

Digestive enzymes for digestion and absorption of foods. Particularly if food allergies or food intolerances are present, in which case, a Biolectrical Impedence Measurement test or an Offsite Cellular Energy Hair Analysis may be performed (see resources)

Parasite remedies

Homeopathics –

Helianthus to support spleen

Apis can clear congested lymph

Lycopodium can clear mucus

Natrum can balance electrolytes

FOODS TO EAT

Manganese – bacterial illness

Potassium – reduce post nasal drip, thin mucous

Magnesium

Zinc – army of immune system

Calcium

EPA/DHA

ADDITIONAL SUGGESTIONS

Swinging

Chiropractic cervical adjustments

Lymphatic massage

Visceral massage

Epsom salt baths ¼ c of Epsom salts in bath water

Ear candling

4 Respiratory System
Description
Support Activities
Toxins to Avoid
Common Nutritional Supplementation
Foods to Consider
Additional Suggestions

Description

The Respiratory system is made up of your not only your lungs, nose, sinuses, mucous membranes, but also the canals to the ears, windpipe and diaphragm. These are the tissues that take in air as it is breathed into the body, remove toxins, keep out air-borne foreign invaders, and cleanse the air to pure oxygen before it enters the circulatory system.

The lungs are the first organ we think of when we think respiratory. They are the largest part of this system, but couldn't do their their job without the partners working with them. They are divided into four quadrants and in our typical hectic day to day breathing, we are typically breathing with the left and right upper first and second quadrants. This is the very definition of shallow breathing, as you will see if you look in a mirror. The neck will 'turtle neck" when one tries to take a deep breath and the shoulders will rise. Try putting a hand on the upper belly and try to push the hand out with breath as breath comes in. Notice in the mirror that you did not raise your shoulders or turtleneck. This is important to make note of, as many lung illnesses end up in these poorly used third and fourth quadrants. These quadrants are also the major avenue for oxygen to enter the bloodstream. This is why, when you feel winded, or dizzy, it is often advised to take deep breaths; to better the chance of oxygen circulating all the way to the brain.

The nose is the cartilage structure that forms the housing for the nasal passages and the beginning of the mucous membranes. The mucous membranes are skin that wraps from the outside into the interior moist environment that makes up the mucous membranes. These membranes are first line defenders in preventing germs and bacteria to the inner workings of our bodies. The sticky mucous traps the offenders and dirt so that you can blow it out of the nose. The tiny hairs inside the nasal passages also protect against dust and dirt.

In ayurvedic medicine it is believed and practiced that the nostrils each are attuned to and energetically associated with the sun and the moon, with warming and cooling, and that these breathing practices need to be incorporated for balance. A Single Nostril Breathing exercise is listed in the Support Activities Section following.

The diaphragm is an important muscle that is kept in shape through a strong core muscle group in the abdomen and the act of breathing. It is like the "windbag" for the body, helping oxygen to be moved all the way through the lungs. Having strong core abdominal muscles is not just for looks and flat abs, but support many functions in the body, including a strong diaphragm.

Support Activities

Breathwork

It is easy to take breathwork for granted because we assume we don't need to as it is an activity we do every day, all day. However, intentional breathing is essential for our health and respiratory support as well as healthy emotions and stress levels.

For 10 minutes in the morning and 10 minutes at night, one should pay particular attention to the breath.

1. At first, just observe. Notice your breath coming and going.
2. Now, Count how long it comes in, how long it is held, and how long it exhales.
3. Try to extend each of those actions by one count and repeat this new count 5 times.
4. Gradually increase your count, and using repetitions of five breaths at each new count, until your time is up.
5. Notice how your whole body feels. Describe it in your mind so you remember the difference between this and your normal breathing.
6. It helps to write these descriptions down so that during the day, when you need to relax, you can pull out your list and your mind will instantly take you back there.

This is an example of one simple breathwork activity. There are many from various practitioners and videos. Find those that feel best for you. Consistent breath practice reminds us that without breath, nothing else exists for us. In that single realization, life changes, as we realize life wouldn't exist without this singular function we take for granted. What else matters?

Diaphragmatic Breathing
Single Nostril Breathing

Did you know? Throughout the day, we predominately breathe through one or the other nostril. Your body regulates your energy and emotional states by switching your dominant nostril every 90 or 150 minutes. You can alter and support your emotional states by breathing through the nostril of your choice. For example, if I am feeling angry and heated, I would plug my right nostril and breathe through my left.

"The right nostril is energetically associated with our body's heating energy, symbolized by the "Sun" and the syllable HA, our left nostril with our body's cooling energy, symbolized by the "Moon" and the syllable THA.

In the average person these energies are typically in conflict, which leads to disquiet and disease. The goal of traditional Hatha Yoga is to integrate and harmonize HA and THA for happiness and health. The purpose of these two breaths then is to create balance by "warming" a "cool" body-mind and vice versa. "[14]

Single Nostril Breathing Techniques
(credit: kundaliniwomen.org)

The following breathing techniques support your mental and emotional balance.
- **Left Nostril Breathing: Relax**
- *Description:* Left nostril breathing activates the *Ida Nerve Ending* in the left nostril, which relates to calmness and relaxation. Left nostril breathing is associated with the moon energy, which is changeable, feminine, yin, giving, and cool. Breathing through the left nostril for five minutes can calm you and lower your blood pressure.

Breath: Sit in Easy Pose. Close your right nostril with your right thumb, your other fingers are stretched straight up as antennas. Your left hand is in Gyan Mudra (illustration) on your left knee. Close your eyes and concentration at your 3rd Eye. Begin to breathe long and deep only through your left nostril. Continue for three minutes.
(Illustration XX)

- **Right Nostril Breathing: Active**
- *Description:* Right nostril breathing activates the *Pingala Nerve Ending* in the right nostril, which relates to alertness and activity. Right nostril breathing is associated with the sun energy, which is a constant, masculine, yang, and hot. Breathing through the right nostril for five minutes can energize yourself and raise your blood pressure.

---

[14] http://www.yogajournal.com/pose/single-nostril-breath/#

Breath: Sit in Easy Pose. Close the left nostril with the left thumb, the other fingers are stretched straight up as antennas. The right hand is in Gyan Mudra (Page XX) on your right knee. Close your eyes and concentrate at your 3rd Eye (Page XX). Begin to breath long and deep only through your right nostril only. Continue for three minutes.
(Illustration turn)

Yogi Tip
When you want to switch your energy, breath through the nostril of your choice.
- **Alternative Nostril Breathing: Balance**

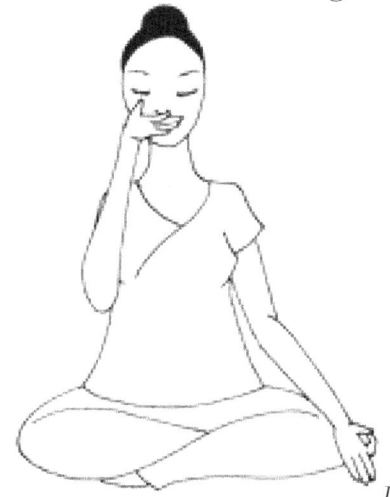

- *Description:* Alternative Nostril Breathing creates a relaxed, harmonious feeling, as it balances the left and right hemispheres of the brain. Practice before bed or when tense.

Breath: Sit in Easy Pose. Your left hand is in Gyan Mudra (Page XX) on your left knee. Close your eyes and focus at your 3rd Eye. Breathe relaxed, deep, and full, as you practice the following sequence, for 3-5 minutes.
- Inhale through the left nostril (Close your right nostril with your right thumb)
- Exhale through your right nostril (Close your left nostril with your right index or ring finger)
- Inhale through your right nostril (Close your left nostril with your right index or ring finger)
- Exhale through your left nostril (Close your right nostril with your thumb)[15]

---

[15] http://kundaliniwomen.org/yoga_pages/yogic_breathing.html

Toxins to Avoid
Chemical fumes
Paint
New furniture off gassing, either delay purchasing, or buy used
Nail Polishes, nail polish remover, hairsprays
It might be time to look into personal care products and make some changes!
Deodorizers and air fresheners, sprays and plug in, as well
Perfumes, colognes
Soaps, detergents, dishwasher mist
Shower heads- keep in mind that chlorinated water is in public water supply and can be breathed in the vapors of a shower. A shower filter might be a good option to purchase.

Common Nutritional Supplementation
Quercetin
Apiol
Echinachea
Vitamin C
Zinc
Probiotics
Mullein
Slippery Elm
Marshmallow Root

Foods to Consider

At this time, mucosal foods and mucus causing foods are a good idea to keep off your plates. The body is producing mucous to protect itself and does so in the amount necessary. Foods like dairy, cheese, sugar, breads are all part of this mucous forming category.

Adding foods that are mucous forming in the body are not encouraged. Eliminative foods, like fruits, vegetables, dark leafy greens are a great option. Be sure to eat quality proteins like beans and chicken turkey or fish, as well as nuts and avocadoes

Additional Suggestions
Singing lessons

Running while singing
Lung breath output devices, like those used after surgery are great to exercise the lungs and surrounding muscles.
Avoid allergic substances, particularly if there is a known allergy. Consider environments and the time of year.
Consider that as the mucous lining of the respiratory is the same tissues as the intestines, care for both systems is a good idea.

When the Respiratory System is Stressed

Personal Journal During Upper Respiratory Infection, Cough, Asthma, Whooping Cough

1. I made an ointment by melting ¼ c coconut oil with 2 cloves of garlic. When the garlic turned brown around the edges, I took it out, removed from heat, cooled and added 5 drops each of Eucalyptus OIl and Peppermint oil. Applied to feet, with socks, chest, back, neck, sinuses. Use repeatedly to maintain a thin layer, I did once per two hours.
2. The pattern and frequency of the description Whooping Cough is cold. Warming oils, blankets, warmth to countermatch. Sunlight, heat lamps, infrared dome, sauna, steam in bathroom - for short amounts of time.
3. I made a marshmallow root tea which is known to be a mucous expectorant with 1 tsp dried marshmallow root in 2 cups water, heated over 15 min. In my 2 year old, I droppered it 5 ml at a time every 15 minutes for three hours. In myself, I would sip throughout the day.
4. Useful herbs: I used 10 drops oregano oil, myrrh, and goldenseal. 3 times daily for adult, half the dose I used for my 2 year old.

5. Hot teas, chicken broth as tolerated, and avoided foods until appetite came back.
6. Lots of rest and fluids. Coffee enemas in those that can
7. As caregiver, I make sure to wash with colloidal silver and take internally along with oregano oil, myself. I continuously cleaned hands and surfaces with colloidal silver or hydrogen peroxide.
8. Outside fresh air in humid warm climates for 15 minutes at a time so as not to tire.
9. Intonation with the challenge frequencies of sounds: ahm ton nah (ahmmm, tone, nahhhhhhh) deep full rich tone. Avoid high pitches.
10. Online users, Click here for the frequency imprint grid pattern.

Common Sense Caution

This is my journal only. Not intended to replace individual health care. For educational purposes only. Please see your health care provider.

5 SKIN
Description
Support Activities
Toxins to Avoid
Common Nutritional Supplementation
Foods to Consider
Additional Suggestions

Description

The skin is an interesting organ in the body. Seen alone, separate from the frame of the body it is an interesting mass of limp coagulant goo, slippery and stretchy. It reminds me of a science experiment as a child in which you would mix a few kitchen compounds together and end up with a stretchy slimy substance that miraculously curls back into itself.

We take for granted that the skin is a huge defender of the body from internal and external attack. Of course we have learned that the skin keeps out unwanted germs from the external world but little attention is paid to the internal defense it puts up. You see, the skin is not just the covering on the outside of the body, but rather, where it meets the few orifice openings into the inner body, it continues on inside, melting and forming itself so that a tube runs from mouth to anus and back outside the body in the form of the skin we see on the outsides of the body. The best way to see this represented is at your mouth. You can touch the skin on of your cheek with your finger, and then follow the skin to the lips and feel that the skin wraps from your lips on into your mouth to form the inner lining of the mouth. This skin is smooth and slick as it has fat and mucosal agents as well as salivary glands, so the feeling is different. This skin runs all the way down your throat, into your stomach, becomes your intestines, and then your rectum eventually out the anus and wrapping around to form the exterior skin of the buttocks.

Taking care of skin on the inside is just as important as taking care of the skin on the outside. Outside, the skin can get ripped, torn, or cut, allowing the potential for foreign invaders to make their way inside the body causing trouble. The same is true for the skin inside. It can get weakened and thin, torn and stretched. In the stomach we know it as ulcers. In the intestines, we know this as leaky gut, allowing "invaders" even though it is simply the things we ingest to now look like bad guys that enter our bloodstream through this now too permeable lining of skin.

Taking care of the skin on the inside is the same as what we do on the outside. Well, with a few changes to conventional primping we have been trained to believe in. For example, conventional lotions. Essentially we are feeding ourselves with whatever that lotion is made up of. Imagine wiping a pile of that pumped out concoction onto your tongue. Do you think your body wants that? Now I know perfumed fragrances and softening creams are all the rage, but to what extent are we damaging not only our skin, but our bodies as a whole?

It is time to go through those personal care cupboards and toss out everything you would not feel comfortable rubbing on the skin of your mouth. Some substitution suggestions are given.

First things first: bathing. Skip the bubbles and body washes. I know it's not as fun but your body will thank you. I always bathe in a bath with a cup of epsom salts. Not only is it detoxifying, but the skin will love to lap up the minerals within. If I am having a particularly acidic outbreak, such as eczema, skin rash, hives, poison ivy or the like, I will add a quarter cup of apple cider vinegar. That's it.

For my face, my regimen is simple. I wash with the water from the bath, then I use freshly squeezed lemon juice as a toner, followed by coconut oil as a moisturizer. For intense moisture and antioxidant detoxification of the skin, I will use a mask of honey and chamomile, but for everyday, I simply use the lemon and coconut oil. The lemon is a toner, firms the skin, lightens freckles and age spots, and smoothes over any wrinkling. The coconut oil is a fantastic moisturizer that doesn't clog pores, is nourishing, and keeps the collagen and elastin underneath the skin well formed.

In case of a pimply breakout, I simply add to the routine a tablespoon of baking powder to just enough colloidal silver water and wash my face with that, which can be used daily. Of course, it is also time to look at the diet at this point, as well.

For sunblock, which I feel is very important, I simply use the coconut oil, which has been scientifically proven as a sunblock. Plus, you'll smell great, and it doesn't feel oily or greasy.

Now, what to do with eczema or psoriasis prone skin. Not only do I follow the above regimen, but here I what I do if I have had a particularly bad episode. Keep in mind, that if eczema or psoriasis are present, it's time to check the diet.

Environmentally Balancing Problem Skin:

Here is what I've done with a severe skin issue that broke out all over my arms, hand, belly very severely.

I cleaned it with smart silver and coconut oil(as the soap).

I washed once daily in the morning and tried to avoid weather and water the rest of the time. I then coated it with olive oil or coconut oil and castor oil, then opened up a cap of activated charcoal, added colloidal silver and dabbed it on the affected areas. This I either left open or cut the toes off a sock and covered my hands so the black wouldn't get everywhere.

I paid attention if it felt too dry then I sprayed on or rubbed on more castor oil. I took 8 capsules of amylase and digestive enzymes internally. I also opened up amylase, mixed in a bowl of water and applied to area by spraying. This can sting though, so I added more water or waited until it was less sensitive. To keep my body strong in case of bacteria, parasites and viruses, and to prevent infection, I took 5 drops oregano oil 3 times a day and a clove of minced garlic at night.

I also did an AIP diet, light exercise and coffee enemas doubled up in both morning and night.

Also, depending on if the skin felt itchy because of dryness, I made moist wraps. I soaked cotton strips in olive oil, wrapped them around my arm and hand, then took a cut up tshirt rectangle and wrapped that around. Lastly, I wrapped in plastic wrap. This would usually alleviate the itch to sleep the night. Sometimes, I did the activated charcoal application, and then wrapped them. This seemed to balance the dry to moist all night long. I could tell when it was time to remove it because the itch returned. At that time, I would clean it with the colloidal silver and coconut oil and bathe the area in a bowl of water with oil and an amylase capsule opened up into it.

Lastly is spiritual transformation that is purely unexplainable. It helped me, and if yourself in the same position, ask yourself what you could be protecting yourself from, what you are irritated by, or what you are being too "permeable" with. What should you say no to? Rest and get to know yourself.

A popular supplement according to Dr. Schulz:
"Researchers have reported that people with eczema do not have the normal ability to process fatty acids, which can result in a deficiency of gamma-linolenic acid (GLA).3 GLA is found in evening primrose oil (EPO), borage oil, and black currant seed oil. Some,4 , 5 , 6 but not all,7 , 8 , 9 , 10 double-blind trials have shown that EPO is useful in the treatment of eczema. An analysis of nine trials reported that the effects for reduced itching were most striking.11 Much of the research uses 12 pills per day; each pill contains 500 mg of EPO, of which 45 mg is GLA."[16]

Supplements to Consider
Slippery elm
Marshmallow root
Chamomile, lavender, and/or lemon verbena tea
Aloe Vera
Vitamin C
Zinc
Iron
Endocrine support supplements
Consider progesterone deficiency.
Omega 3's
Vitamin E
Vitamin K

Foods to Add
Iodine rich foods
Kelp
Dulse
Nori
Seaweed

---

[16] Dr. Schulze's Incurables

Gomasio
Essential fatty acid foods
Healthy fats
Avocado
Leafy Greens
Foods containing GLA

Additional Tips
The skin will reflect whatever is going on internally. Both physically and emotionally.
Skin is heavily reliant upon the liver health, so be sure to read the section on liver and bowels. The liver is heavily influential on hormone health and the skin will be a direct reflection of this health or lack thereof. So talk to your provider about hormone imbalance.It is also going to be the last system in the body to receive nutrients, so talk to a nutritionist or nourishmentalist or record for yourself to be sure you are getting enough nutrients, and also that you are digesting and absorbing what you do take in, to be sure the skin is receiving the food it needs.

Be Gentle on your skin. Skin naturally sloughs off its own dead skin with mild gentle help from our fingers or soft rag. Don't use harsh abrasives or chemical soaps.

6 Emotions

Description
Support Activities
Toxins to Avoid
Common Nutritional Supplementation
Foods to Consider
Additional Suggestion

Description

It's no longer a surprise to hear people talk about emotions and their fair share of health troubles. I believe the health of the body is greatly made up of what we have imprinted onto it with our thoughts, words, beliefs, ideals, and attitudes, including how much fun we have in our life.

I believe our individual outer worlds are a direct expression of our inner beliefs and how we present ourselves and our lives out into the world.

I also believe what a professor told me years ago. He said, "If you let a person speak long enough, eventually they will tell you what's wrong with them." And this really is where it begins, and treatment should start here. Because this is what is on the person's mind. Lay the person open like an onion, letting the layers fall apart as they will and soon you will see the core, but the trick is to handle the layers as they drop.

Though all of these are certainly not indicative of your concerns, it is a starting place to look into what is going on with the emotional systems of the body and how they may be playing into the symptoms expressed by the body. Look at them for reference, but look further, asking yourself when the last time the particular system was normal and what could have been a trigger.

Liver and Bowel:

Guilt
Inadequacy
Self-rejection
Doubt
Anger
Bitterness
Regret
Resisting what IS
Control
Not going with the flow of life
Strict with self and others
Judgemental
Self Worth
Victim mentality
Lack Mentality
Not being able to digest life
Type A personality
Balance of yes to no, wrong to right, work to play, control to acceptance

Kidney and Bladder:

Not going with the flow
Fear
Control
Holding on
Not letting go
Disappointment
Failure
Shame
Fear of Death
Childhood issues
Issues with parents learned as a child
Sexual beliefs

Lymphatic:

Lack of willpower
Lack of self confidence
Not good enough
Needs courage
Resentment
Stubbornness
Revenge (seem to cause the diaphragm to shift upward blocking lymphatic movement)

Lung:

Strong
In Charge
Dominant
Don't breathe the breath of life
Control
The Illusion of Power
Trouble with Authority
Trouble with God and divinity
Taking time for oneself

Skin:

Being too permeable
Being too compliant
Being not permeable enough
Holding things in
Closed or too open
Can't say no
Sensitive
Imbalance
Tenderness, gentleness
Issues with self, aloneness, oneness
Fear of being touched

Support Activities
Journal
Find a good listener
Seek out a good counselor
Do things that make you happy and make you YOU

Read into material on emotionally based health problems
Read on metaphysical meaning
Feel your emotions don't deny them, but do it in a safe way, for you and others.

Toxins to Avoid
A toxic physical body will wreak havoc on the spiritual and emotional bodies, so keep the body clean and healthy.
Avoid preservatives, dyes, food colorings
Maintain a healthy diet to avoid GMOS and chemicals
In addition, change your life to avoid toxic people, situations, toxic talk and thoughts about yourself.
Avoid foods that don't honor life.

Common Supplementation:
ALL nutrients and a healthy diet are important for emotional, psychic, and spiritual health. Find a good supplemental regimen that's right for you.

Bach Flowers - "The original Bach Flower Remedies is a safe and natural method of healing discovered by Dr. Bach from 1920 – 1930's in England. They gently restore the balance between mind and body by casting out negative emotions such as fear, worry, hatred and indecision which interfere with the equilibrium of the being as a whole. The Bach Flower Remedies allow peace and happiness to return to the sufferer so that the body is free to heal itself.
The Bach Flower Remedies are made from wild flowers and are safe for the whole family including pets."[17]

Foods to Add
Foods that serve and honor life
Foods that make you feel healthy rather than weigh you down
Foods that have psychological meaning for you need to be removed from the diet, and then added back in after dealing with the trauma they are associated with.

---

[17] http://www.bachflower.com/original-bach-flower-remedies/

A Final Note

Your body is the only vehicle you have to perform your work while you are here. Your direct enjoyment of the experiences of your life are affected by the health of your body. It is wise to keep the body clean and in balance so that you can assist it in it's functions, thus avoiding costly and debilitating illnesses and disease. But even more so than avoiding disease, care of your body is important so that you can live a life you want to live.

Complete Resource Listing

Find natural health practitioners in your area:
http://www.mnanp.org/
http://www.naturopathic.org/af_memberdirectory.asp?version=2
https://mn.gov/boards/medical-practice/public/find-practitioner/
www.thenaturalsourcecompany.com
www.theextremepotential.com

Offsite Cellular Energy Testing(through hair analysis):
Comprehensive Health Technologies
healthhelp@live.com
320-250-9072

Bioelectrical Impedence Measurement Testing:
www.thenaturalsourcecompany.com
www.iht-bio.com

LIVER AND BOWELS SYSTEM RESOURCES

Supplementation:
www.nut-dyn.com for supplementation
Ultra dophilus, ultra flora spectrum, Spectrazyme digestive enzymes, silymarin, milk thistle

Probiotics:
www.nut-dyn.com , Ultraflora varieties
http://www.lucyskitchenshop.com/acidophilus.html, acidophilus
https://www.natren.com/probiotic-supplements.html, Natren company probiotics, for powdered varieties

Enema bags:
http://www.vitalitymedical.com/enema-bag-sets-with-slide-clamp.html?gclid=Cj0KEQjwzZe8BRDguN3cmOr4_dgBEiQAijjVFnFrYwsCEfQYyf0Ze7J4NolYVmqLl3ezHRCa4Y5a4m8aAtFT8P8HAQ

Yogurt Maker:
http://www.lucyskitchenshop.com/yogourmet.html

Yogurt Starter/Fermented Foods starter:
http://www.lucyskitchenshop.com/yogourmet.html#starter

Castor oil pack kits:
http://www.radiantlifecatalog.com/product/premier-castor-oil/superfoods-supplements/?a=96418

Herb orders:
http://www.radiantlifecatalog.com/
https://www.mountainroseherbs.com/

Anti-Inflammatory Diets:
http://thepaleodiet.com/, paleo diet
www.theextremepotential.com, digestive help, IByes protocol
"No Grain, No Pain", by Amanda Plevell
http://www.gapsdiet.com/, GAPS diet
http://www.breakingtheviciouscycle.info/, SCD diet
http://pecanbread.com/, Kids on the SCD
http://www.thepaleomom.com/the-autoimmune-protocol/, AIP

Research Further:
Dr. Josh Axe
Dr. Mercola
Bernard Jensen
Gerson Miracle
Pinterest recipes by peers

KIDNEY/BLADDER SYSTEM RESOURCES

www.nut-dyn.com for nutritional supplementation

Overworked Kidneys Supplements:
https://www.swansonvitamins.com/HealthConcern/Kidney+Health

Azo Cranberry:
http://www.azoproducts.com/products?gclid=Cj0KEQjwztG8BRCJgseTvZLctr8BEiQAA_kBDytd706F3u6JGhK6URAe073NafAFd41RaGnhODrvIJsaAtMV8P8HAQ

LYMPHATIC SYSTEM RESOURCES

dry skin brushes:
http://www.amazon.com/gp/offer-listing/B00BAZ4P4G/ref=asc_df_B00BAZ4P4G3015198?ie=UTF8&condition=new&tag=pgmp-681-97-20&creative=395169&creativeASIN=B00BAZ4P4G&linkCode=asm

loofah sponges:
http://www.amazon.com/AquaBella-5-5in-Loofah-Body-Twin/dp/B001CTUMTM/ref=sr_1_3?ie=UTF8&qid=1393631922&sr=8-3&keywords=loofah+mitt

coconut oil(for post dry skin brushing):

http://www.amazon.com/Barleans-Organic-Virgin-Coconut-16-Ounce/dp/B002VLZ8D0/ref=sr_1_4?s=hpc&ie=UTF8&qid=1393631999&sr=1-4&keywords=coconut+oil

sunflower oil (for post dry skin brushing and oil pulling):
http://smudeoil.com/

crystal body deodorant:

http://www.amazon.com/Crystal-Stick-Body-Deodorant-sticks/dp/B000L978FU/ref=sr_1_1?s=hpc&ie=UTF8&qid=1393633489&sr=1-1&keywords=crystal+deodorant

non aluminum cookware:
http://www.amazon.com/Cook-Home-NC-00358-Nonstick-PTFE-PFOA-Cadmium/dp/B00FM9QZXA/ref=sr_1_9?s=home-garden&ie=UTF8&qid=1393633553&sr=1-9&keywords=non+aluminum+cookware

non aluminum baking powder:
http://www.amazon.com/Bobs-Red-Mill-Double-Aluminum/dp/B005P0I7T6/ref=sr_1_1?s=grocery&ie=UTF8&qid=1393633630&sr=1-1&keywords=non+aluminum+baking+powder

spry toothpaste:
http://www.amazon.com/Xlear-Spry-Toothpaste-Flouride-toothpaste/dp/B000LRI6J4/ref=sr_1_1?s=hpc&ie=UTF8&qid=1393633678&sr=1-1&keywords=spry+toothpaste

Supplements:
www.nut-dyn.com
Advaclear, UltrClear Plus PH detoxification
UltraPotent C, Sinuplex, Nazanol for sinus and lymphatic

RESPIRATORY RESOURCES

http://www.yogajournal.com/pose/single-nostril-breath/

Shower filters:
http://www.homedepot.com/p/High-Output-3-Spray-4-in-Fixed-Shower-Head-with-Filter-in-White-HO2-WH-M/100372129

SKIN SYSTEM RESOURCES

Activated Charcoal:
http://earthshiftproducts.com/Products/Supplements/cleansing-and-detox/ACTCHA/CHARPOW4

EMOTIONS RESOURCES

Concept pathology:
www.theextremepotential.com, CPT technique, CPT appointment, Success Conditioning exercises and books

Concept Therapy:
http://www.concept-therapy.org/, The Concept Therapy Institute
Dr. Thurman Fleet
Dr. Jason Lupkes, Lupkes Family Chiropractic, St. Cloud, MN
"Rays of the Dawn"

Bach Flower Remedies:
www.thenaturalsourcecompany.com, consulting appointment
www.theextremepotential.com, remote appointment
http://www.bachflower.com/original-bach-flower-remedies/, to purchase remedies

Emotions and healing:
Lousie Hay and the Hay House
"You Can Heal Yourself", Louise Hay
"What to Say When you Talk to Yourself"
https://www.amazon.com/What-Say-When-Talk-Yourself/dp/0671708821

References

http://www.livestrong.com/article/184493-how-to-dry-brush-your-skin/

http://www.oilpulling.com/

Baker, Joyce, *Computerized Electrodermal Screening", p.24*

http://www.yogajournal.com/pose/single-nostril-breath/

http://kundaliniwomen.org/yoga_pages/yogic_breathing.html

Dr Schulze's Incurables http://healingtools.tripod.com/incurprog1.html

Prostaglandin, role of food, herbs, blockers www.raysahelian.com

Natural Non-Drug Remedies for Inflammation www.drmhaatma.com
Reducing Inflammation with Diet and Supplements: The Story of Eicosanoid Inhibition www.itmonline.org

How to Naturally Lower Prostaglandins With Foods LIVESTRONG.COM www.livestrong.com

Natural Remedies - Part 1: Supplements and Herbs for the Relief of Pain, Swelling and Inflammation
www.cascadewellnessclinic.com

http://wellnessmama.com/35671/castor-oil-packs/

http://enzymedica.com/blogs/digest-this/15843160-health-benefits-of-enzymes

http://www.scdiet.org/2recipes/scdyogurt.html

"The WHYs behind the Autoimmune Protocol: Nightshades", Foods in Moderation, The WHYs of the AIP by ThePaleoMom

https://www.merckmanuals.com/professional/genitourinary-disorders/tubulointerstitial-diseases/heavy-metal-nephropathy

http://www.webmd.com/vitamins-supplements/condition-1536-Renal+failure.aspx

https://www.swansonvitamins.com/HealthConcern/Kidney+Health

http://www.bachflower.com/original-bach-flower-remedies/

http://kathyhadleylifecoach.com/spiritual-causes-of-diseases/

ABOUT THE AUTHOR

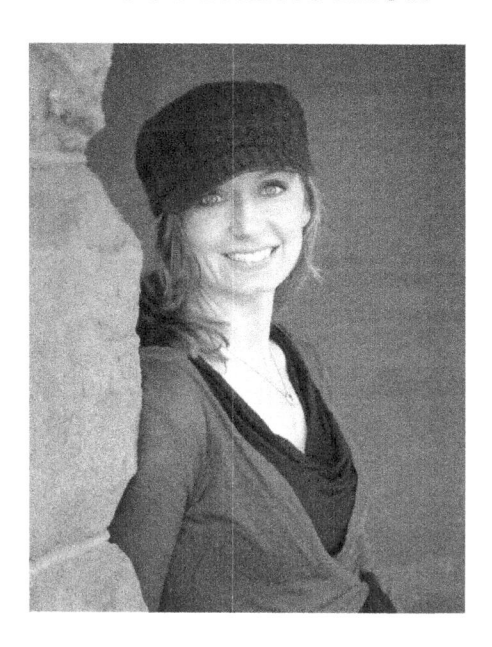

Soulvay (Amanda) Plevell, CNHP, is an Author and Educator, speaker and trainer on the inspiring topics of naturalism and natural wellness. She is the founder of The Natural Source Centers and theextremepotential.com, which are missions working to serve mass consciousness by helping people to improve their lives by providing resources. Visit her at her websites:
www.thenaturalsourcecompany.com
and www.theextremepotential.com
and follow her on facebook.

Made in the USA
Monee, IL
02 July 2021